Body Safety Education

A parents' guide to protecting kids from sexual abuse

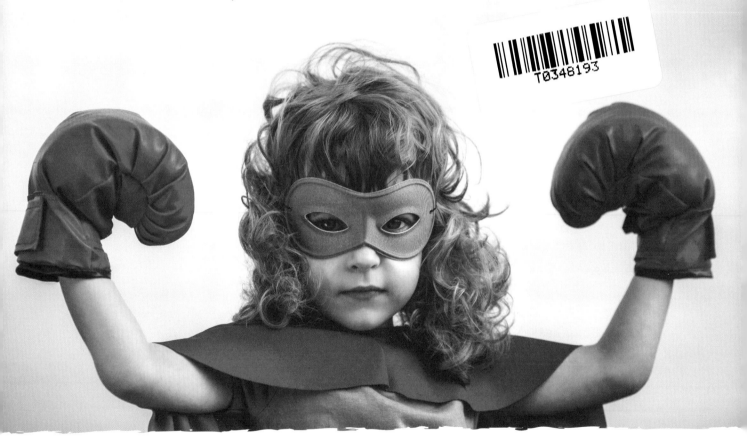

by Jayneen Sanders

Body Safety Education
Educate2Empower Publishing an imprint of
UpLoad Publishing Pty Ltd
Victoria, Australia
www.upload.com.au

First published in 2015
Reprinted in 2018

Written by Jayneen Sanders

Jayneen Sanders asserts her right to be identified as the author of this work.

Designed by Ben Galpin

Printed in China through Book Production Solutions

ISBN: 9781925089394 (hbk)   9780987186089 (pbk)

A catalogue record for this book is available from the National Library of Australia

Acknowledgments
Cover and p1: © Sunny studio/Shutterstock.com; p4: © AtthameeNi/Shutterstock.com; p5: © Nolte Lourens/Shutterstock.com; p7: © altanaka/Shutterstock.com; p8: © Blaj Gabriel/Shutterstock.com; p10 and p47 (Illustration-white hand on black): © gst/Shutterstock.com; p13: © Denis Kuvaev/Shutterstock.com; pp15, 50, 51 (Illustration): © Matthew Cole/Shutterstock.com; p16: © Sergiy Bykhunenko/Shutterstock.com; p18: © Angela Waye/Shutterstock.com; p20: © Gladskikh Tatiana/Shutterstock.com; p21: © fasphotographic/Shutterstock.com; p22: © AnikaNes/Shutterstock.com; p24: © RimDream/Shutterstock.com; p26: © Alexander Trinitatov/Shutterstock.com; p27: © altanaka/Shutterstock.com; p29: © Shestakoff/Shutterstock.com; p30: © Blend Images/Shutterstock.com; p32 (left to right): © Sunny studio/Shutterstock.com; © fasphotographic/Shutterstock.com; p33: © Kamira/Shutterstock.com; All illustrations unless otherwise specified by Cherie Zamazing

Disclaimer: The information in this book is advice only written by the author based on her advocacy in this area, and her experience working with children as a classroom teacher and mother. The information is not meant to be a substitute for professional services or advice. For professional help if you are concerned about a child's behaviour, go to a health professional and/or contact the Key Organizations listed on p. 37.

Contents

Introduction

Child sexual abuse statistics are confronting. Approximately 20% of girls, and 8% of boys will experience sexual abuse before their 18th birthday (*Pereda, et al, 2009*). What is equally terrifying is that in approximately 85% of child sexual abuse cases, the child will know the offender (*NSW Commission for Children & Young People, 2009*). The abuser will most likely be a close family member, a family friend or some one the child comes into contact with regularly. The perpetrator is rarely a stranger.

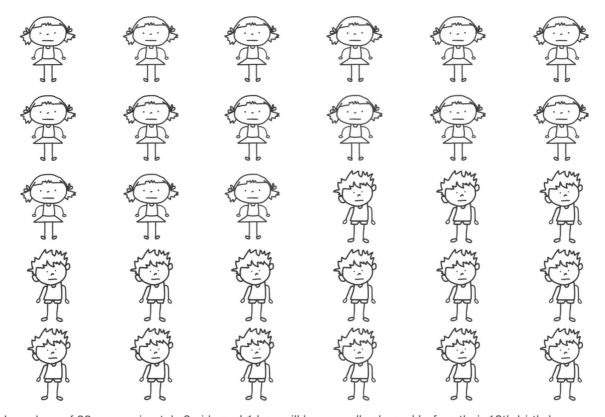

In a class of 30, approximately 3 girls and 1 boy will be sexually abused before their 18th birthday.

Child sexual abusers are in our community and they are in our homes. They can be anyone. As parents, educators and community members, it's time to act. We need to empower the children in our care through Body Safety Education. The effects and the incidences of childhood sexual abuse can be greatly reduced through preventative education and community awareness.

> *'Child sexual abuse is about the abuse of power.*
> *It involves the strong and well-informed using the powerless*
> *and uninformed for sexual pleasure and degradation.'*

From *Teaching Children to Protect Themselves* by Professor Freda Briggs, Allen & Unwin, 2000

What Is Body Safety Education?

Body Safety Education (aka sexual abuse prevention education) aims to empower children with skills and knowledge that will lessen the likelihood of them becoming victims of childhood sexual abuse.

In summary, Body Safety Education teaches children:

- the correct names for their private body parts
- the difference between safe and unsafe touch
- not to keep secrets that make them feel bad/uncomfortable
- what to do if they are touched inappropriately
- general assertiveness — especially in relation to their own body.

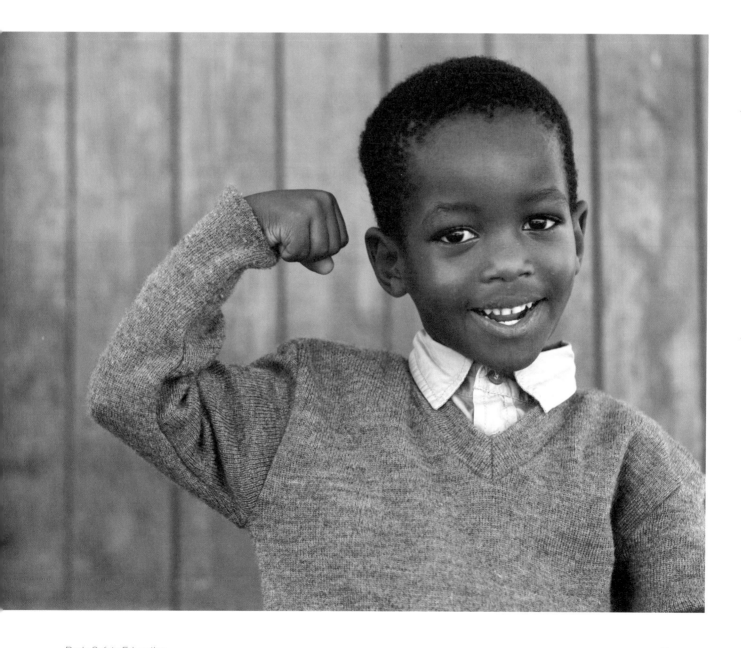

Why Is It Important to Teach Children Body Safety?

It is natural we want to protect the children in our care and to keep them 'safe' at all times. While we can control their environment to some extent, we can't be with them every minute of every day. At some stage in their young lives, they will have to go out into the world without us. The world is not always a pleasant place, and sadly in the interests of our children, we must face up to the following facts:

1. The sexual abuse of children has no social boundaries. Predators come from all racial, ethnic, religious, economic and educational backgrounds. Similarly, children from any of these groups can be and are targeted by sexual predators.

2. 85% of children who are sexually abused will know the offender (*NSW Commission for Children & Young People, 2009*). The abuser will most often be someone they know and trust.

3. Perpetrators 'groom' both the child and the family, and prey upon both in order to achieve their goal, which is to sexually abuse the child.

4. Up to 95% of child sexual abusers are male (*Bagley, 1995*). They can be single, married and have families of their own.

5. Up to 1/3 of reported offenses are committed by adolescents (*Bagley, 1995*). More and more we are seeing cases of child-on-child sexual abuse, and older children/siblings sexually abusing younger children.

6. The most vulnerable age for children to be exposed to sexual abuse is between 3 and 8 years with the majority of onset happening between these ages (*Browne & Lynch, 1994*).

The consequences of childhood sexual abuse are devastating both to the survivor and their families. A survivor, more often than not, has ongoing health issues such as anxiety, depression, eating disorders, drug and alcohol abuse, post-traumatic stress syndrome as well as trust, security, confidence and relationship issues.

It has also been documented that survivors of childhood sexual abuse are 10 to 13 times more likely to attempt suicide (*Plunkett et al, 2001*). The effects of childhood sexual abuse can be intergenerational. Children of survivors may live with a parent who has ongoing mental and physical health issues that, in turn, can affect their own well-being and that of their children.

We cannot let our adult fear of this topic put our children at risk. We have a duty of care to teach children their rights in regards to their body. So many survivors of childhood sexual abuse say — if only they had known 'it' was wrong. And this is where Body Safety Education comes in — an educated child will know, from the first inappropriate touch, that it is wrong and they will know to tell and keep on telling until they are believed.

NOTE

As a community, we have a duty of care to believe children and not dismiss their disclosures as 'untrue' simply because the act of a child being sexually abused is so abhorrent to us, and therefore it couldn't possibly be true. See p. 26.

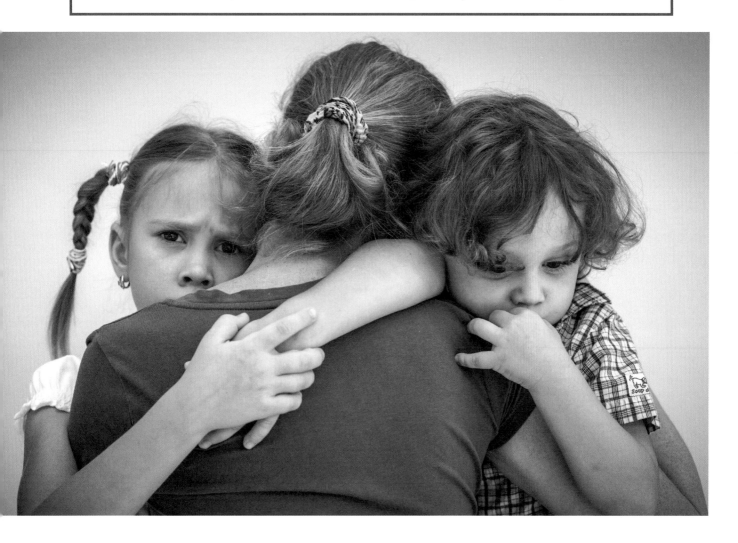

Key Body Safety Skills

The following Key Body Safety Skills should be taught gradually and in daily conversations as your child grows. If you are concerned about teaching your child these skills, just keep in mind they are age-appropriate, non-graphic, and they also encourage your child to be assertive — a crucial skill in any bullying situation, and a great attribute to have when your child becomes a teenager!

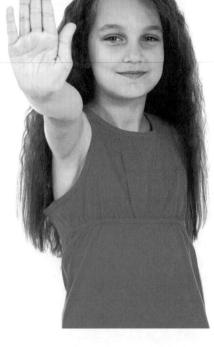

1 **As soon as your child** begins to talk and is aware of their body parts, begin to name them correctly, e.g. toes, nose, eyes, arms, legs, etc. Children should equally know the correct names for their genitals from a young age. Teach your child that their penis, vagina, vulva, bottom/buttocks, breasts and nipples are called their 'private parts', and that these are their body parts under their swimsuit. Try not to use 'pet names'. This way, if a child is touched inappropriately, they can clearly state to you or a trusted adult where they have been touched. A child's mouth is also known as a 'private zone'. (Resource Masters 1–6 can be used to identify private body parts and teach that private body parts are those under a child's swimsuit.)

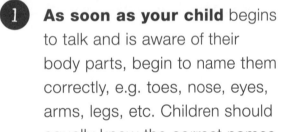
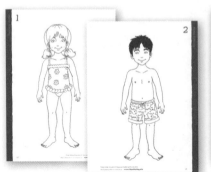
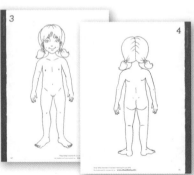
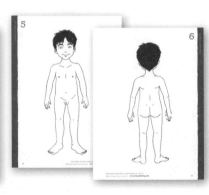

2 **Teach your child** about boundaries from a young age. Use the idea of a 'bubble' around them approximately the size of a hula hoop. Refer to this bubble as their own personal space that no one has the right to enter if they don't wish them to. Let your child know they have the right to say 'No!' if someone does enter their personal space/bubble/body boundary. They also have the right to say 'No' to being kissed or hugged by another child, an older child/teenager or an adult. The older people in your child's life also need to respect your child's boundaries and their wishes. Moving on from this, don't force your child to show affection if they don't wish to by making them kiss or hug another person. This only reinforces to your child that their wishes don't 'really' matter. In order not to insult the older person, your child could simply shake hands or give a high-five this time around. Learning about consent is crucial for a young child and importantly transfers into their teenage and adult years. People in your child's world need to understand that when your child says 'No' (especially in relation to their body) they mean 'No'. This needs to be respected and adhered to.

Now might be a good time to introduce the concept of 'private' and 'public' places. Briefly talk about a 'private' place as the toilet or bathroom (even their bedroom as they get older) and a public space as an area used and shared by everyone. The idea behind this concept is that children understand that when they go to the toilet or have a shower they have the right to privacy. People should never walk in on a child (or anyone) in a private space, and if someone does, they should tell a trusted adult straightaway. Of course, if your child is very young, they may need help with toileting and showering, and they may share a bedroom with siblings so the idea of 'private' and 'public' places can be tricky. However, it is still important that they know people must always seek their consent before entering a private place. It is also important to note as part of the grooming process, predators may walk in on children showering and/or toileting so as to 'normalise' this behaviour. However, a child who is educated to understand the difference between a 'private' place and a 'public' place will also know to tell a trusted adult if anyone does this to them. The line between 'private' and 'public' places will become less blurred as children get older and become more independent.

3 **Teach your child** that no one has the right to touch or ask to see their private parts, and if someone does, they have the right to yell 'No!' or 'Stop!' They should then quickly move away and tell a trusted adult. Reinforce that they must keep on telling until they are believed. Statistics tell us that a child will need to tell three people before they are believed. Educate your child that if someone (i.e. the perpetrator) asks them to touch their own private parts, shows their private parts to the child or shows them images of private parts (pornography/child exploitation material) that this is wrong also, and that they must get away quickly and tell a trusted adult. Ensure your child knows that they are the 'boss of their body' and if an older person does touch their private parts, they are never to blame. It is very empowering for children to physically practice placing their hand out in front of them, standing firm and tall, and saying in a loud strong voice: a) 'No!' or b) 'Stop!' or c) (in a bullying situation) 'I don't like that!' or d) 'Stop! I am the boss of my body!' Throughout your child's life continue to reinforce this concept.

NOTE

The perpetrator may show the intended victim child exploitation material to convince him or her that such acts are 'normal' and therefore permissible. See p. 29.

---

4 **As your child becomes older** (3+ years) assist them to identify three to five trusted adults (one should be from outside the family) who they could tell if they are touched on their private parts, asked to touch someone's private parts or are shown inappropriate images.

NOTE

Ask the people your child nominates if it is okay for them to be on your child's network — I suspect they will be honoured; if they are not, than they are not the right people to be included on your child's safety network!

The three to five people nominated by your child are part of their 'safety network'. Have your child point to each digit on their hand and say the names of the people on their safety network. Another great idea is to draw an outline of your child's hand (or make a handprint with paint) and label each digit with the name of their safety network person. Your child could draw a picture of that person at the end of each digit or you could paste on a photograph (for children not yet reading). Display their safety network hand in a prominent place. Resource Master 7 could be used as an alternative to outlining your child's hand. Resource Master 8 is a sample letter you may wish to give to those people who have regular contact with your child. The letter informs them that your child is educated in Body Safety, and asks them to be a part of this ongoing and important education.

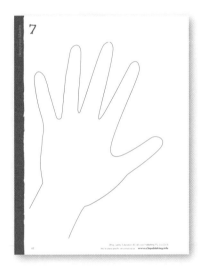 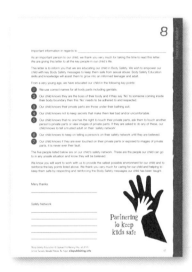

NOTE

Some children may want to add their pet or toy to their safety network. This is okay. They can be added to the palm. However, reinforce gently to your child that the pet/toy is great to tell about an unsafe situation but they won't be able to do anything; and that they will also need to tell a trusted adult who can actually help them.

---

5. **Talk about feelings** with your child at the same time as you are discussing inappropriate touch. Discuss what it feels like to be happy, sad, angry, excited, etc. Use posters (see the *Body Safety and Respectful Relationships Teacher's Resource Kit* at **www.e2epublishing.info**) or story books to talk about how the child on the poster or in the story book might be feeling. During daily activities, encourage your child to talk about their own feelings,

e.g. 'I felt really sad when … pushed me over. I felt really scared on the big slide. I felt happy when Bec asked me to play with her.' This way your child will be more able to verbalize how they are feeling if someone does touch them inappropriately. Resource Master 14 and the children's book *Talking About Feelings* (**www.e2epublishing.info**) could both be used to help children explore their feelings.

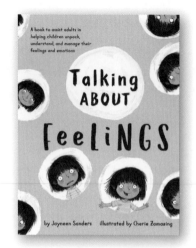

6 **Talk with your child** about feeling 'safe' and 'unsafe'. This is a concept young children find hard to grasp. Discuss times when your child might feel 'unsafe', e.g. being pushed down a steep slide; or 'safe', e.g. snuggled up on the couch reading a book with you. Children need to understand the different emotions that come with feeling 'safe' and 'unsafe'. For example, when feeling 'safe', they may feel happy and have a warm feeling inside; when feeling 'unsafe', they may feel scared and have a sick feeling in their tummy. Allow your child time to verbalize how their body reacts when they feel 'safe' or 'unsafe'. The cards from the Teacher's Resource Kit can be used for this activity and are available at **www.e2epublishing.info**

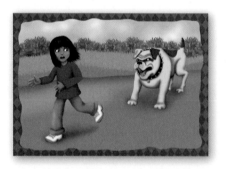
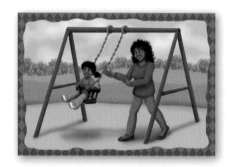

7 **When in an unsafe situation** we all experience our 'early warning signs'. These are the messages our body sends to us when we feel unsafe. Discuss with your child their early warning signs, e.g. heart beating fast or hard, feeling sick in the tummy, sweaty palms, feeling like crying, weak or shaky legs. Let them come up with some ideas of their own. You could use Resource Master 9 to label your child's early warning signs. Tell your child that they must tell you or a trusted adult on their safety network if any of

Body Safety Education

their early warning signs happen in any situation. Reinforce that you (and the people on their safety network) will always believe them and that they can tell you anything.

8   **As your child grows**, try as much as possible to discourage the keeping of secrets. Talk about 'safe/happy surprises' such as not telling Granny about her surprise birthday party and 'unsafe/bad' secrets such as someone touching their private parts. Make sure your child knows that if someone does ask them to keep a secret about inappropriate touching or viewing images of private parts that they must tell you or someone on their safety network straightaway.

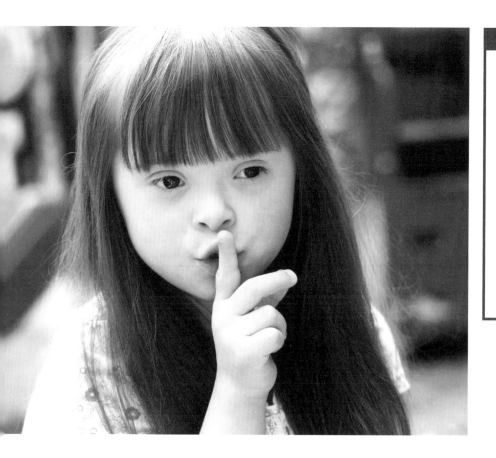

NOTE

The keeping of secrets is a crucial part of the grooming process used by perpetrators (see p. 17) and therefore it is **very important** your child knows the difference between happy surprises and a secret that makes them feel bad and uncomfortable.

9   **Discuss with your child** when it is appropriate for someone to touch their private parts, e.g. a doctor when they are sick (but making sure they know you or a person from their safety network must be in the room). Discuss with your child that if someone does touch their private parts (without you there) that they have the right to say 'No!' or 'Stop!' and outstretch their arm and hand, then get away as quickly as possible and tell a trusted adult. Children (from a very young age) need to know their body is their body and no one has the right to touch it inappropriately.

10 **Read the children's books** *No Means No!*, *My Body! What I Say Goes!*, *Some Secrets Should Never Be Kept* and *Let's Talk About Body Boundaries, Consent and Respect* with your child regularly. The discussion questions at the back of each book are invaluable for the all-important and ongoing discussions with your child. Go to **www.e2epublishing.info** for more information on how to purchase these resources. Educate2Empower Publishing also offers many free posters, songs and videos; please go to the website and explore further.

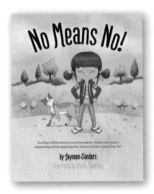 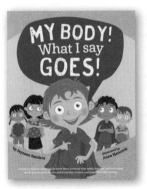 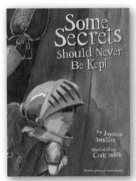 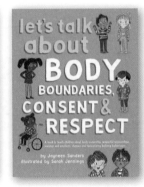

11 **Continue to reinforce** the Body Safety message by trying some 'What could you do?' scenarios with your child. You can use this time to talk about all sorts of emotional issues as well as Body Safety scenarios.

For example:
- What could you do if someone took your bucket and spade from the sandbox?
- What could you say/do if you didn't feel like a goodbye kiss from Grandpa?
- What could you do if another child asked to see your private parts?
- What could you do if an older person touched your private parts or asked you to touch theirs?
- What could you do if someone pushed you down the slide?
- What could you do if a child at school showed you their private parts?
- What could you do if a person asked to see your private parts?

Make up your own scenarios to suit your child and the discussion/s you wish to have. Ask yourself, What learning do I want my child to achieve from this discussion? See also Body Safety Skills Conversation Starter Cards on pp. 54–63.

Lastly, sexual abuse prevention education is not only a parent's responsibility, it is also the community's responsibility. Ask your child's child-care centre, kindergarten or primary/elementary school if they are running a Body Safety program. If they are not, ask why not. And **please** lobby for it. See Educating the Community on p. 31.

NOTE

Educating your child in Body Safety may not only protect them, but it may protect other children as well. It is not uncommon for children to disclose sexual abuse to a friend. The friend needs to know that what happened to the child who disclosed is wrong and they must tell a trusted adult immediately — even if the other child has asked them to keep it a secret.

Be Proud

Be proud (and loud) that you educate your child in Body Safety. Your child should also be proud that they are educated in Body Safety. There are two very good reasons for this:

1 Body Safety knowledge empowers children. It goes a long way in keeping them safe from sexual abuse, and ensuring they grow up as assertive and confident teenagers and adults.

2 Talking openly and proudly that your child is educated in Body Safety, and that there are no secrets in your family, sends a clear message to potential perpetrators that your child will not become one of their victims, and that they can no longer hide behind the community's fear and silence on this once-taboo subject. (Use Resource Masters 11, 12 and/or 13 [colouring-in sheet] and display in a prominent position.)

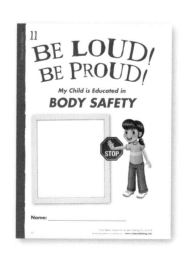

Final Tips

1. There is no 'special time' to teach Body Safety. It needs to be an ongoing and natural discussion as your child grows. It is best to relax and make the discussion as casual and informal as possible, using 'teachable moments' when they arise. For example, when your child is old enough to wash and dry themselves when bathing, ask them to wash and dry their own private parts. This is a good time to reinforce that their body is their body and only they can touch it. By creating a home environment where there is openness, discussion and no topic is 'off the table', it will be much easier for your child to talk to you if something does happen. If you are tense and uptight, your child will take these cues from you and think these 'conversations' may be something to worry about — which of course they are not!

2. Talk about and ensure you child has a sound understanding of public and private places/ spaces. For example, you could say that public places are 'shared by everyone' such as the lounge room in the house and the playground at school; but private places are 'just for you' such as the toilet/bathroom and our bedroom. Point out if someone wants to enter our bedroom they should ask us if it is okay as it is a private place.

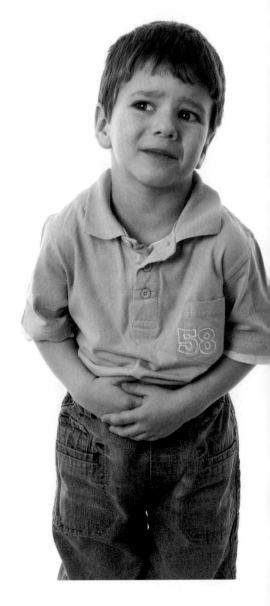

3. Trust your child. Just like adults, children have an 'inbuilt radar' when it comes to safe and unsafe touch. If they say they don't want to go with someone or they don't want to be left alone with a person (who you may even deem a good friend), trust your child's instincts and respect their wishes.

4. For some children (particularly boys) the inappropriate touch of the perpetrator may feel pleasurable. Therefore, it is imperative when educating children that they know their private parts should not be touched even it feels good.

Grooming and Awareness

Grooming, in order to sexually abuse a child, is about establishing power over that child, and using that power to maintain the secret. It is about making sure the child never tells. Grooming can take place over days, weeks or years. A groomer taking time to 'groom' enables trust between themselves and the child (and the family) to build up. This trust, in turn, creates opportunities for regular abuse to occur. Force is rarely used but rather emotional coercion. An abuser uses their power to exploit the child's trust and innocence.

Be aware of:

1 Any person who wishes to spend a great deal of time with your child, seeking out their company and offering to take care of them at any time. For example, an abuser will often 'help out' the targeted family at short notice, appearing as a reliable and trustworthy friend. This is the persona a sexual predator will go to great lengths to establish, enabling them to spend more time alone with your child without suspicion.

2 Any person who pays special attention to your child, making them feel more special than any other child; providing them with special treats, presents, candy, etc. These 'treats' may be provided without your knowledge and be the first of your child's secrets they are being groomed to keep. The child will be made to feel as if they are the groomer's 'confidant'.

'The strategies employed by offenders to gain the compliance of children more often involve giving gifts, lavishing attention and attempting to form emotional bonds than making threats or engaging in physical coercion. Many sexual encounters with children were proceeded by some form of non-sexual physical contact.'

(Smallbone & Wortley, 2000)

3 Any person who spends a large percentage of their out-of-hours recreation time with children — often without other adults present or preferring to be 'alone' with the children.

> **NOTE**
>
> In saying this, of course we want our children to spend quality and loving time with the special adults in their lives. However, it is important to stay alert!

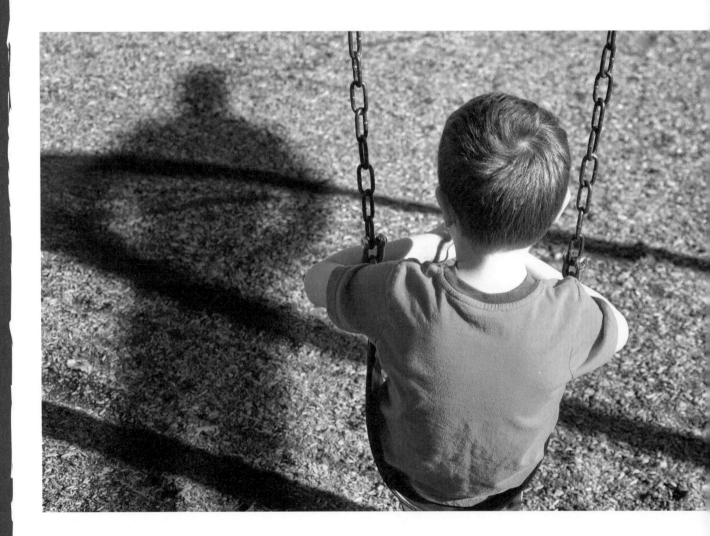

Important Things to Know About Abusers

Child sexual abuse is a crime and punishable by law. Child sexual abusers are skilled at deception and conniving in all their perverse undertakings. They will:

1   **Always** plan their sexual abuse of a child. In fact, they may plan and 'groom' for a number of years before making sexual contact with the child. They will plan in detail how they will spend time with the family and the child, how they will get time alone with the child, and especially what threats they will use on the child in order for the abuse not to be revealed. Ensuring the child 'keeps the secret' is of extreme importance to the offender — if the child does tell, the consequences for the offender are catastrophic. Therefore, they will use whatever means they can for the child to keep the secret. This includes subtly discrediting the child by making them out to be a liar — so if they ever do disclose, they won't be believed.

2   **Choose** a victim very carefully. They will test the child's reaction to physical touch such as rubbing the child's shoulder or an arm, or stroking his or her hair and then watching for the child's reaction. If the child is receptive, the touching will continue. The touching may well start out as an 'innocent', 'fun' game of tickling that the child enjoys, but later when the abuser deems the child 'groomed', the touch will turn to sexualized contact.

NOTE

Adult/older child rough-housing, tickling, wrestling and any kinds of hands-on play are often fun for kids. However, if the play is most often initiated by the adult/older child, involves a lot of body touching and the person doesn't stop when the child asks them too; observe that person carefully. Grooming involves blurring the lines between what is appropriate/fun touch and inappropriate touch. This blurring confuses a child into believing they were a willing participant in the inevitable sexual contact. Of course we want to have fun with our kids and physical play is part of that, but if a child says 'No' and that they have had enough, we need to respect their wishes. This respect for 'No' carries through into adulthood via teenage-hood!

3 **Encourage** the child to keep secrets that at first may not be of a sexual nature. These 'fun secrets' are intended to build up a sense that the abuser and the child have a 'special' relationship. These 'fun secrets' will turn to secrets of a sexual nature once the perpetrator deems the child 'ready'.

4 **Coerce** the victim into believing the sexual abuse is 'normal', 'love-based' and/or the child's idea. They will use 'guilt', 'shaming' and 'blaming' techniques to convince the child into believing that they are an equal participant in the 'shameful' secret, and therefore are equally to blame. The child can be so 'guilt ridden' that they may never disclose. This is particularly relevant to young boys who may find the touch pleasurable, and this only leads further to their confusion. The perpetrator will use these feelings to their 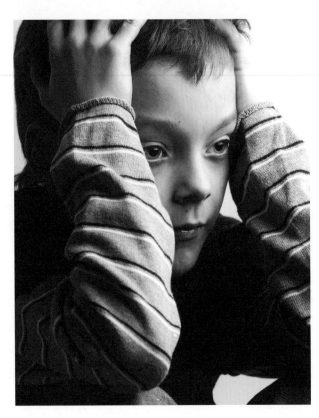 advantage, noting that the child responded to the touch and 'liked it', thereby reinforcing the idea that they are a willing participant in the 'secret'. Never underestimate the devious and manipulative nature of a sexual predator.

5 **Use** threats and blackmail to ensure the child keeps the secret — threats such as the child will go to jail if they tell and that they will never see their family again, that no one will believe them and that they will destroy the family, etc. The abuser will work very hard to ensure the child never tells, and they will always make the child feel that they are to blame.

NOTE

It is crucial that children are taught not to keep secrets that make them feel bad and/or uncomfortable. Secrets and threats are the currency sexual predators use to stay hidden.

Body Safety Education

6 **Work** very hard at being liked (even loved) by the child and his or her family. For example, the abuser will often help the family out on short notice, appearing as a reliable and trustworthy friend. This is the persona the abuser will go to great lengths to establish.

7 **Scheme** to get 'alone time' with a child (or group of children) and will spend a lot of their out-of-hours recreation time with children.

'Because the offender is often a person well-known and trusted by the child and their family, they usually can easily arrange to be alone with the child — therefore the abuse is commonly repeated. This abuse rarely involves violence because instead of force, these offenders use promises, threats and bribes to take advantage of their trusted relationship with the child's family and the subsequent powerlessness of the child. In some cases, this can go on for years.'

(NSW Child Protection Council, 2000)

8 **Target** busy parents who are in need of extra help. They will also target vulnerable and disadvantage communities.

'Children who live with a single parent that has a live-in partner are at the highest risk: they are 20 times more likely to be victims of sexual abuse than children living with both biological parents.'

(Sedlack et al, 2010)

9 **Change** jobs and addresses frequently to avoid detection.

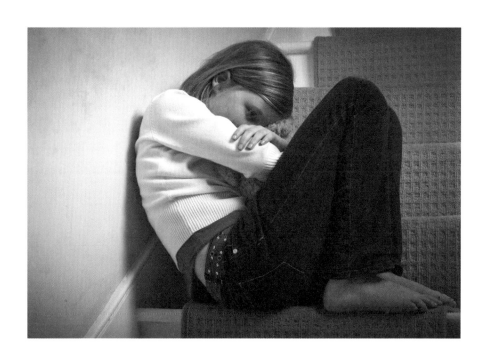

What Is Normal Sexual Behaviour?

Sex is a normal part of life and naturally children are curious about it. They wonder about the physical differences between boys and girls, where babies come from and what the many oblique references to sexual behaviour are all about. They will experiment from an early age and role-play what they have seen no matter what the source. It is difficult for parents to know what is 'normal' and expected in their behaviours. 'Normal' is a very problematic word and there can be no hard and fast rules. The following guidelines are just that, guidelines. If your child falls outside these parameters it is not necessarily indicative of a problem, but if you are concerned you should discuss it with a child-care professional. Try not to react in a negative way to age-appropriate sexual behaviours. Sexual curiosity is how children learn about who they are.

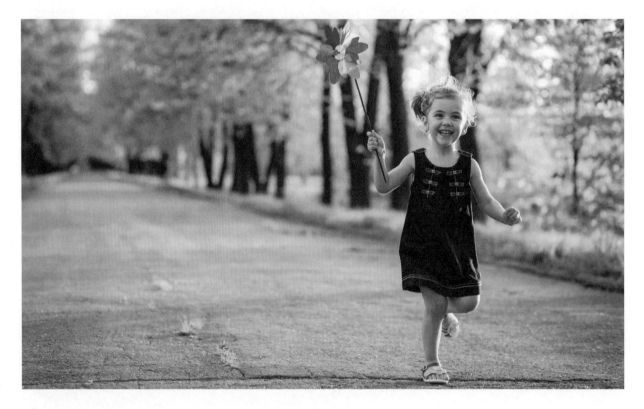

Some examples of age-appropriate sexual behaviours are:
- babies, toddlers and young children exploring their genitals and enjoying being naked
- questions about why they have a penis and girls don't (and vice versa), i.e. trying to work out the difference between what it is to be male and what it is to be female
- showing others their genitals

- playing doctors and nurses and/or mothers and fathers; kissing or holding hands with children of a similar age
- using slang words or 'rude' words they have picked up
- looking at each other's body parts (particularly children: under 7, close in age and those who know each other) in mutual agreement, i.e. no one is being forced to show each other their body parts

- as they get older, being curious about where they came from; may be giggly and embarrassed about body-parts discussions

General Signs of Sexual Abuse

A child who is being sexually abused may show a number of telltale signs of the abuse (see list below.) However, it is important to also note, a child may drop subtle hints such as acting up when the abuser is about, or feeling sick when it's time to go to the abuser's home — consciously or subconsciously hoping someone will 'pick up' on these indicators. Children who are being sexually abused are, in most cases, too scared to actually tell their crippling secret, so it is crucial we maintain our parent/teacher 'radar' for the subtle signs a child may be trying to give us.

In Children 0 to 12 Years

- overly interested in theirs or other's genitals
- continually wants to touch private parts of other children
- compares genital size with older children
- instigating and/or forcing 'sex play' with another child (often younger, more than 3 years difference in age)
- inappropriate sex play, e.g. oral-genital contact between a 7 year old and a 4 year old (note: with the increase in pornography viewing on the internet by young children, sex play is becoming more worrisome among similar-aged children)

- inappropriate sex play with another child happening more than 3 times, despite careful monitoring and discussion about inappropriateness
- persistent masturbation that does not cease when told to stop
- seductive/advanced sexual behaviour
- sexualized play with dolls or toys or animals
- sexualized play involving forced penetration of objects vaginally or anally
- chronic peeping, exposing and verbalizing obscenities
- touching or rubbing against the genitals of adults or children that they do not know
- persistent use of 'dirty' words
- describing sexual acts and sexualized behaviour beyond their years
- drawings and/or games that involve inappropriate sexual activities
- drawings that include large genitals on naked or clothed bodies
- becoming upset when viewed changing clothes
- talking in a sexualized way with unknown adults or older children
- strong body odour
- sores around the mouth
- bruising, scratches, rashes, cuts, burns or bleeding in the genital area and/or breasts, buttocks, lower abdomen or thighs
- blood or discharge on sheets or in underwear
- pain while urinating or with bowel movements
- frequent urinary tract infections
- withdrawn and anxious behaviour (irritable, clingy, listless)
- excessive crying and unable to be soothed
- secretive or say they have a 'special' secret they can't tell (this may be to gauge your reaction)
- child or child's friend telling you about interference directly or indirectly
- going to bed fully clothed
- increase in nightmares and sleep disturbances

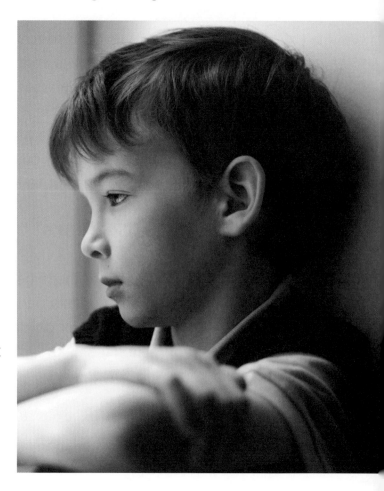

- regressive behaviour, e.g. a return to bed-wetting or soiling
- sudden changes in behaviour, e.g. from a happy child to an angry and/or defiant child
- learning difficulties, poor concentration, lower grades, problems with peers (however, some children are the perfect student)
- appetite changes (sudden and significant), failure to thrive
- unexplained accumulation of money and gifts
- increased talk of a 'special older friend'
- may show increase in delinquent behaviour (most likely 8 years and above)
- not wanting to go to a certain person's place or to an activity
- indirectly dropping hints about the abuse (again, to gauge your reaction)

In Older Children (Adolescents)

Please note: adolescents may also display some of the indicators on pp. 23 to 25.

- self-destructive behaviour such as drug and/or alcohol dependency, suicide attempts, self-mutilation
- eating disorders
- delinquent behaviour such as stealing, lying and vandalism
- ticks, phobias, obsessions
- persistent running away from home and/or refusal to attend school
- withdrawal from family and friends
- increase in angry/aggressive behaviour
- low self-esteem statements such as 'I deserve to be dead'
- saying that their body is dirty, ruined, damaged
- overly modest when changing or showering around others on camp or school sports
- verbalizing sexually aggressive obscenities
- secretive about their 'special friends' on the internet/in their life
- suspicious of people, not allowing anyone to get physically or emotionally close
- adolescent pregnancy
- sexually promiscuous (having multiple partners from a young age; sometimes much older partners)
- performing sex for money
- fear of sexual intimacy

- overly interested in pornography
- presence of a sexually transmitted infection

One or more of these indicators does not mean a child is being sexually abused, but if they do show some of these indicators, then there is good reason to investigate further.

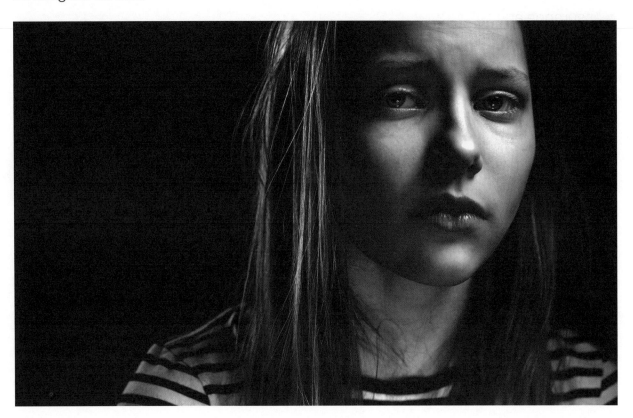

Disclosure and the Importance of Believing a Child

It cannot be reinforced strongly enough how important it is to believe a child if they disclose sexual abuse. In 98% of reported child sexual abuse cases, children's statements were found to be true (*NSW Child Protection Council, cited in Dympna House, 1998*). Our reaction to a child's disclosure is crucial to their ongoing well-being and healing. If we react with disbelief, they may never tell again and their suffering will only increase; they may also let the abuse continue. If we react with shock, horror and/or anger, the child will most certainly take their cues from us, and believe that in some way they are to blame. It takes an enormous amount of courage for a child (or adult) to disclose sexual abuse that may have been ongoing for years.

They may have been threatened with horrific consequences were they to tell, or it could be simply that the child was told that no one would ever believe them. Each case is different and most often there are layers of emotional complexities involved. For a child to find the bravery to overcome threats and emotional blackmail is a true act of courage. But what a child needs more than anything from the person they disclose to — be it a parent, relative, teacher or friend — is compassionate reassurance and to be believed. Therefore, stay calm, try not to act emotionally, and:

- reassure the child you believe them
- reassure the child they have done the right thing in telling
- reassure the child that they are incredibly brave and courageous
- reassure the child that they are in **no** way to blame
- reassure the child that they are loved
- reassure the child that they are safe and will be looked after
- reassure the child that you will do everything you can to stop the abuse (however, make no promises)
- once the child is with a trusted and caring adult, contact one of the Key Organizations listed on p. 37 for further advice.

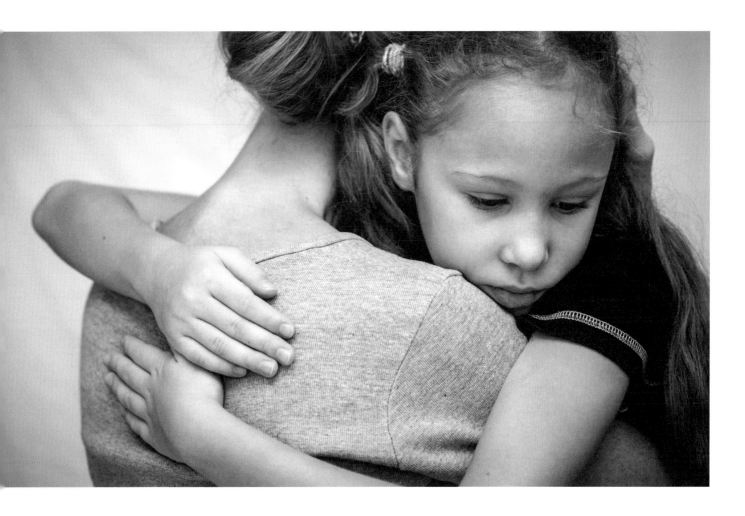

It is our responsibility and duty of care to the child to remain calm as well as receptive and compassionate once he or she begins to disclose. If they disclose amongst a group, take the child aside and find a safe place for them to continue. A disclosure from any sexual abuse victim takes an enormous amount of courage — so please, as the trusted recipient, respond to such bravery with kindness and compassion.

NOTE

If a child begins to disclose abuse amongst a large group, e.g. in a playgroup, a teaching group or when reading Body Safety children's books to a group of children, stop them gently and say, 'What you are going to tell me is very important. We can talk about this after our lesson.' Ensure they know you are concerned and value what they are about to reveal. If another trusted person is available, have them continue the lesson and take the child aside so they can disclose in a safe environment. Protective interrupting is important so confidentiality is kept and it prevents other children from hearing the disclosure. If a child does disclose, see p. 37 and contact one of the organizations listed. They will inform you on how best to proceed.

Many adult survivors say that the most hurtful thing to happen to them when they disclosed, either as a child or adult, was being treated as the offender, and the perpetrator as the victim, e.g. by having a family member say such things as, 'Look what you have done! You have ruined …'s life. He/she will never be the same again.' These examples were actually how one family reacted to a survivor's disclosure and how they aligned themselves with the perpetrator. This kind of reaction is incredibly damaging for the person who has disclosed, and can reinforce the unwarranted guilt and shame that they may well already be feeling. All guilt and shame remains with the perpetrator and they are 100% responsible for the abuse; this is important to remember if a child/ adult does disclose. The survivor needs our support.

NOTE

When adult survivors were asked what is the one thing that could have made all the difference to them as an abused child, the answer was overwhelmingly to be believed.

Internet Pornography and Its Effects

The increased internet usage by younger and younger children provides societal challenges. One of these challenges is that children may be exposed to adult pornography and/or child exploitation material. As part of our ongoing parenting conversation, we need to establish a trusting relationship with our child where they will come to us if they have

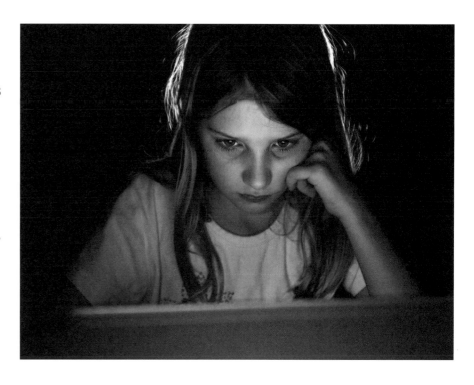

seen or heard anything disturbing. Our relationship needs to be open and honest, and this needs to begin from a young age.

Internet pornography, in relationship to Body Safety Education, raises two main issues:

1 Your child may be exposed to adult pornography and/or child exploitation material by chance, by their own undertaking or by a friend.

2 Your child may be exposed to adult pornography and/or child exploitation material by a sexual predator or an older child.

In both cases, your child needs to be educated from a young age to tell what they have seen (see point 3, p. 9) and who showed these images to them. With an open and honest dialogue with your child, they will know they are not to blame for this exposure. If your child has been exposed to pornographic images, I recommend counselling by a child-care professional.

Links Between Child Sexual Abusers and Pornography

1 Some initial research studies do indicate that child sexual abusers will view pornography with their victims. After the initial grooming of the child (and their family) they will show the child sex acts to normalize the behaviour, and in some cases, arouse sexual curiosity. And, as is the case with all predators, use that curiosity to lay blame on the victim's shoulders.

2 Men, women and teenagers who watch child exploitation material on screen could have an increased danger of acting out what they see; whereas, if they were not exposed to such crimes, they may not have offended against a child.

> **NOTE**
>
> In my opinion, there should be no term 'child pornography' as it is a criminal sex act against a child or children, and is a crime scene. Those viewing it are partaking in a criminal act.

3 Groomers online may expose teens to pornography in order to arouse sexual curiosity and encourage them to meet for sexual acts.

4 Older siblings exposed to internet pornography may (please note, this is a 'may') act out what they have seen on younger siblings who they have ready access to.

5 Anecdotally, educators and health professionals are saying more and more that younger children are acting out inappropriate sexual acts on same-age peers. This could be due to exposure to pornography.

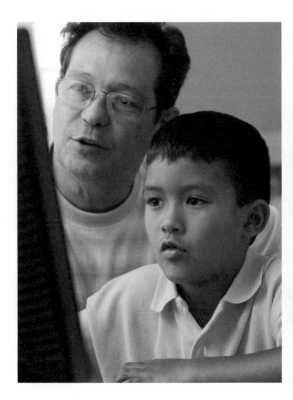

Age-appropriate sex education for our children is paramount, so pre-adolescent children and teenagers don't turn to internet pornography as the only readily available source of information on sex. Unfortunately, what they are seeing by viewing pornography are distorted and disturbing images of what sex and sexual relationships entail.

As parents, we need to be vigilant about our children's use of the internet. Let's make sure we have open and honest discussions with our children and teach them age-appropriate sex education. See p. 37 for links to sex education resources for parents.

Educating the Community

Teaching children Body Safety needs to be a normal part of our parenting conversation. There are a number of reasons for this:

1 To reduce the statistics of child sexual abuse and therefore reduce the ongoing trauma that most often accompanies childhood sexual abuse.

2 To empower our children with knowledge in regards to their body and their right to be safe.

3 To show sexual predators that no longer can they hide behind society's fear of this topic, and we **will** educate our children to tell of inappropriate touch and/or secrets.

Community members need to know that as parents and educators we are proud to provide this knowledge to children in order to keep them safe from sexual abuse. The community has to also be educated to believe a child when they disclose such abuse.

Some time ago I was told this story:

A little girl disclosed to her teacher that she had been sexually abused by her father. She was told by the teacher to sit on the school step and stay there for lying and she was never to tell such terrible lies again. Of course, that little girl never told another person and grew up to be an adult believing she was to blame for the shameful secret, and suffered all the mental and emotional health consequences that this entailed.

No longer can we let our children suffer alone, as we turn the other way. It is time to educate children, parents, educators and the community in Body Safety. With that education comes an added responsibility on the community's part to believe children when they do disclose.

Please feel free to download posters at **www.e2epublishing.info/posters** (see examples below). These free posters can be shared with friends, family and colleagues on social media sites. They can also be printed and displayed at schools or child-care centres. It is up to all of us to educate our community to make this world a safer place for children. I like to call it the 'parent-ripple effect', i.e. by sharing information on Body Safety Education with just one other person/parent, you may actually change a child's life.

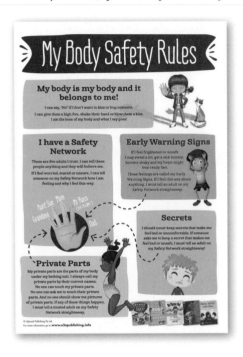
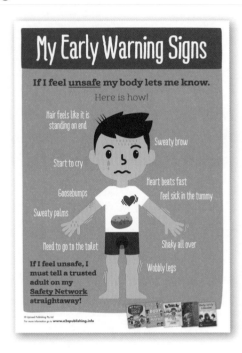

Some Troubling Statistics

1 Approximately 20% of girls, and 8% of boys will experience sexual abuse before their 18th birthday (*Pereda, et al, 2009*).

2 In approximately 85% of child sexual abuse cases, the child will know the offender (*NSW Commission for Children & Young People, 2009*).

3 84% of sexual victimization of children under 12 occurs in a residence (*Snyder, 2000*).

4 The most vulnerable age for children to be exposed to sexual assault is between 3 and 8 years with the majority of onset happening between these ages (*Browne & Lynch, 1994*).

5   20% of women had experienced childhood sexual abuse, with the age of abuse being under the age of 12 years for 71% of these women *(Fleming, 1997).*

6   In 98% of child abuse cases reported to officials, children's statements were found to be true *(NSW Child Protection Council, cited in Dympna House 1998).*

7   1 in 3 Australians would not believe a child if they disclosed sexual abuse *(Australian Childhood Foundation, 2010).*

8   73% of child victims do not tell anyone about the abuse for at least 1 year. 45% do not tell anyone for 5 years. Some never disclose *(Broman-Fulks et al, 2007).*

9   As high as 81% of men and women in psychiatric hospitals with a variety of mental illness diagnoses have experienced physical and/or sexual abuse. 67% of these men and women were abused as children *(Jacobson & Richardson, 1987).*

10   Survivors of childhood sexual abuse are 10 to 13 times more likely to attempt suicide *(Plunkett A, O'Toole B, Swanston H, Oates RK, Shrimpton S, Parkinson P 2001).*

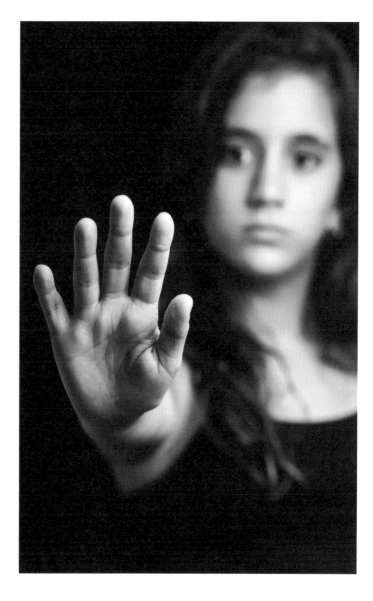

Common Concerns and Questions

1 **My child will lose their innocence if I teach them Body Safety.**
They won't. They will be empowered through knowledge. This knowledge will keep them safe. It is far better that your child is educated than have their childhood stolen. Childhood sexual abuse cannot be undone. Research tells us there is no 'one size fits all' to describe the effects of childhood trauma, but reduced quality of life is a constant.

2 **Sex and the act of sexual abuse will be discussed.**
When we teach road safety to children, we don't show graphic images. Why would we? We are teaching children. Similarly, when we teach Body Safety, all messages are age-appropriate and non-threatening. Sex and the act of sexual abuse is never mentioned.

3 **My child is too young to be educated in Body Safety.**
Three to 8 years is the most likely age for a child to be sexually abused. See p. 32. The younger you start to educate your child the better! As soon as they begin to talk — start!

4 **'Stranger Danger' education is all my child needs.**
Approximately 85% of sex abusers are known to the child. See p. 32. They will be a trusted family member, close family friend, coach, neighbour, etc. Predators are amongst us and they can be anyone.

5 **Why bring up this topic when my child will never be sexually abused?**
Approximately 20% of girls and 8% of boys will experience sexual abuse before their 18th birthday. See p. 32. Chances are your child is more likely to be sexually abused than break a limb. The sexual abuse of children has no social boundaries.

6 **My child doesn't need to be educated in Body Safety; they tell me everything.**
A child can be so threatened and terrified to keep 'the secret' they may never tell. 73% of child victims do not tell in the first year, 45% do not tell in the first 5 years and many never disclose. See p. 33.

7 **I don't want to scare my child.**
All Body Safety Education is age-appropriate and non-threatening. Such education is designed to empower children not to frighten them.

8 **My child is never left alone with other adults.**
Children can be sexually abused by older children and more recently by children of the same age. Research is beginning to show a correlation between a child's exposure to internet pornography and the acting out of sexual acts on same-age or younger children.

9 **My child won't want to hug or show affection to the adults in their life.**
Just like adults children have an 'inbuilt radar'. Through age-appropriate Body Safety Education children learn to recognize safe and unsafe touch and feelings. A child knows when a hug is loving and safe, and when it may feel uncomfortable and wrong. Children educated in Body Safety learn to act upon their unsafe feelings — termed 'early warning signs'. See point 7, p. 12.

Top 12 Children's Books to Keep Kids Safe from Sexual Abuse

There are a number of fantastic books available to teach children Body Safety skills. Children are visual learners so story is an excellent medium when broaching this subject with your child.

1 'My Body! What I Say Goes!' written by Jayneen Sanders, illustrated by Anna Hancock, published by Educate2Empower Publishing 2016

2 'Some Secrets Should Never Be Kept' written by Jayneen Sanders, illustrated by Craig Smith, published by Educate2Empower Publishing 2011

3 'My Body Belongs to Me' written by Jill Starishevsky, illustrated by Sara Muller, published by Free Spirit Publishing 2014

4 'My Body Belongs to Me from My Head to My Toes' created by pro familia, illustrated by Dagmar, published by Sky Pony Press 2014

5 'Everyone's Got a Bottom' written by Tess Rowley, illustrated by Jodi Edwards, published by Family Planning Queensland 2007

6 'The Swimsuit Lesson' written by Joh Holsten, illustrated by Scott Freeman, published by Holsten Books 2011

7 'Matilda Learns a Valuable Lesson' written by Holly-ann Martin, illustrated by Marilyn Fahie, published by Safe4Kids 2011

8 'Amazing You' written by Dr Gail Saltz, illustrated by Lynne Avril Cravath, published by Penguin 2005

9 'The Right Touch' written by Sandy Kleven, illustrated by Jody Bergsma, published by Illumination Arts 1997

10 'I Said No!' written by Zack and Kimberly King, illustrated by Sue Rama, published by Boulden Publishing 2008

11 'No Secrets Between Us' written by Rose Morrisroe, illustrated by Matthew Fox, published by www.nosecretsbetweenus.com

12 'Jasmine's Butterflies' written by Justine O'Malley, illustrated by Carey Lawrence, published by Protective Behaviours WA

'No Means No!' and 'Let's Talk About Body Boundaries, Consent and Respect' are also important books to empower children and teach them about personal boundaries and consent; and are ideal as an introduction to Body Safety Education.

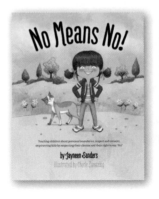
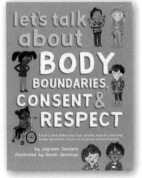

Key Organizations and Important Links

RAINN (US) www.rainn.org

Childhelp (US) www.childhelp.org

National Children's Alliance (US) www.nationalchildrensalliance.org

Darkness to Light (US) www.d2l.org

NSPCC (UK) www.nspcc.org.uk

Stop It Now! (UK) www.stopitnow.org.uk

1800RESPECT (Australia) www.1800respect.org.au

CASA (Australia) www.casa.org.au

Child Wise (Australia) www.childwise.org.au

Australian Childhood Foundation www.childhood.org.au

Bravehearts (Australia) www.bravehearts.org.au

Policelink (Australia) 131 444

See **www.e2epublishing.info** for further children's books, teaching packs; free posters, resources and videos.

See **www.safe4kids.com.au** for a comprehensive Protective Behaviours resource and education programs in Protective Behaviours.

See **www.husheducation.com.au** for information on sex education and Protective Behaviour programs and resources.

See **sexedrescue.com** for a range of books and resources to teach children and adolescents sex education.

See **www.talkingthetalksexed.com.au** for information on sex education and Protective Behaviour programs and resources.

FINAL NOTE

As a brave survivor said to me:

'The more light we shine on child sexual abuse, the fewer shadows there are for abusers to hide in.'

By educating your child in Body Safety you are empowering them with important knowledge and skills. You are also giving abusers fewer shadows to hide in! And for this, I personally thank you!

Jayneen Sanders

About the Author

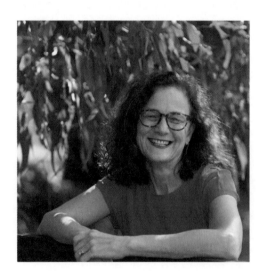

Jayneen Sanders (aka Jay Dale) is an experienced teacher, author, and a passionate advocate for providing all children with Body Safety and Respectful Relationships Education. Her children's books cover Body Safety, consent, gender equality, respectful relationships, and social and emotional intelligence. Jayneen believes empowering children from an early age makes for empowered teenagers and adults. She is also Lead Author for the children's literacy series 'Engage Literacy' published by Capstone Classroom, and has written over 120 titles for that series. As a mother of three, Jayneen has always advocated for children's rights and encouraged them to have a voice. Her ongoing passion for the safety and empowerment of children continues today with new manuscripts and additional free-to-download resources always in the wings. Her work can be found at www.e2epublishing.info and on Amazon.

References

Abel, G. (1994). *National Institute of Health Survey*

Australian Childhood Foundation (2010). *Doing Nothing Hurts*. Ringwood [Vic]: Australian Childhood Foundation.

Bagley, C. (1995). *Child Sexual Abuse and Mental Health in Adolescents and Adults.*

Broman-Fulks, J. J., Ruggiero, K. J., Hanson, R. F., Smith, D. W., Resnick, H. S., Kilpatrick, D. G., & Saunders, B. E. (2007). *Sexual assault disclosure in relation to adolescent mental health. Results from the National Survey of Adolescents*. Journal of Clinical Child and Adolescent Psychology, 36: 260–266

Browne, K. & Lynch, M. (1994). *Prevention: Actions speak louder than words*. Child Abuse Review, 3: 241–244.

Child Protection Council (1993). *Fact Sheet No. 5*. Sydney [NSW]: Sexual Assault Committee.

Dympna House (1998). Info Kit: *A booklet on childhood sexual abuse.* Haberfield [NSW]: Dympna House.

Fleming, J. (1997). *Prevalence of childhood sexual abuse in a community sample of Australian women*. Medical Journal of Australia, 16: 65–68.

Jacobson, A., & Richardson, B. (1987). *Assault Experiences of 100 Psychiatric Inpatients: Evidence of the Need for Routine Inquiry*. American Journal of Psychiatry, 144: 908–913

NSW Child Protection Council, (1998). *Managing Sex Offenders*

NSW Child Protection Council (2000). *Child Sexual Assault: How to talk to children*

NSW Commission for Children & Young People (2009).

Pereda, Guilera, Forns & Gomez-Benito (2009) *The prevalence of child sexual abuse in community and student samples: a meta-analysis.*

Plunkett, A., O'Toole, B., Swanston, H., Oates, R.K., Shrimpton, S., Parkinson, P. (2001) *Suicide risk following child sexual abuse.*

Sedlak, A.J., Mettenburg, J., Basena, M., Petta, I., McPherson, K., Greene, A., & Li, S. (2010). *Fourth National Incidence Study of Child Abuse and Neglect (NIS–4): Report to Congress, Executive Summary*. Washington, DC: U.S. Department of Health and Human Services, Administration for Children and Families.

Smallbone, S. & Wortley, R. (2000). *Child sexual abuse in Queensland: Offender characteristics and modus operandi*. Brisbane [Qld]: Queensland Crime Commission

Snyder, H. N. (2000). *Sexual assault of young children as reported to law enforcement: Victim, incident, and offender characteristics*. Washington, DC: U.S. Department of Justice, Office of Justice Programs, Bureau of Justice Statistics.

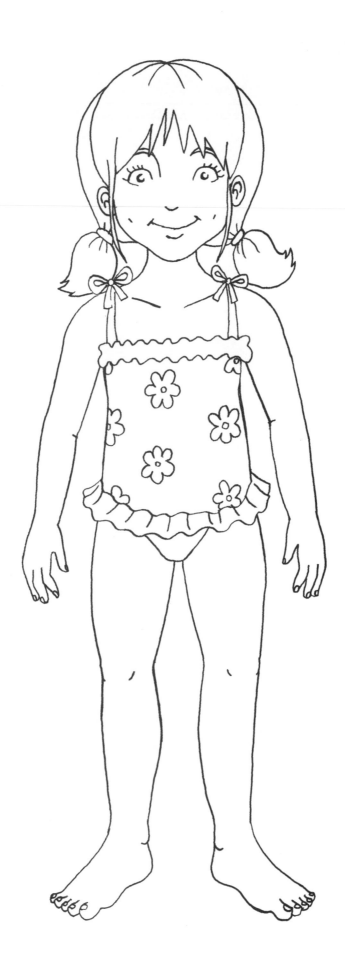

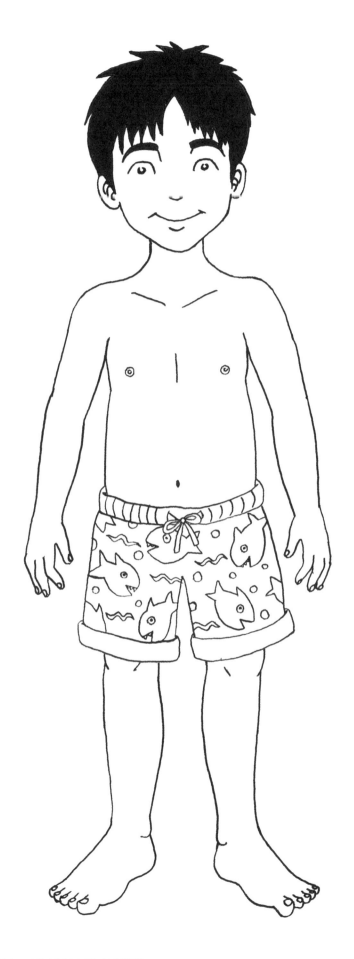

3

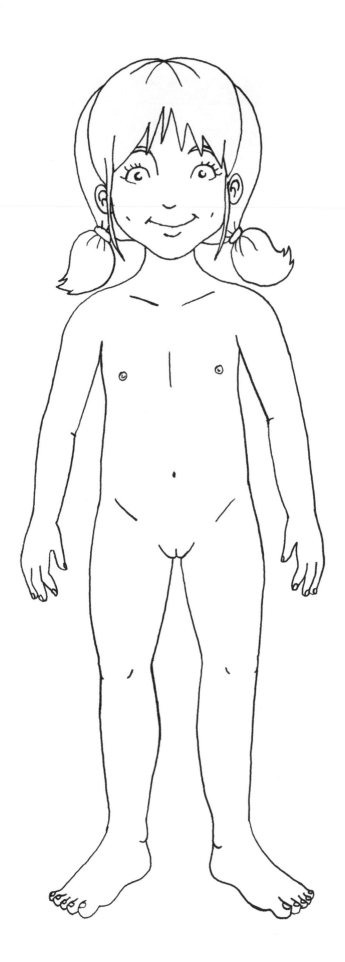

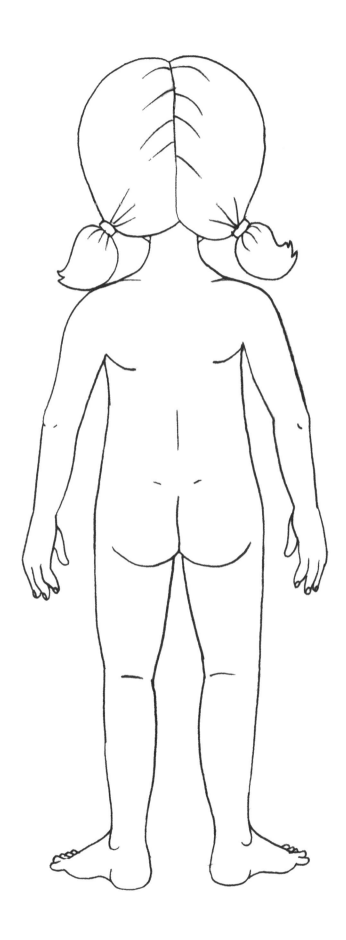

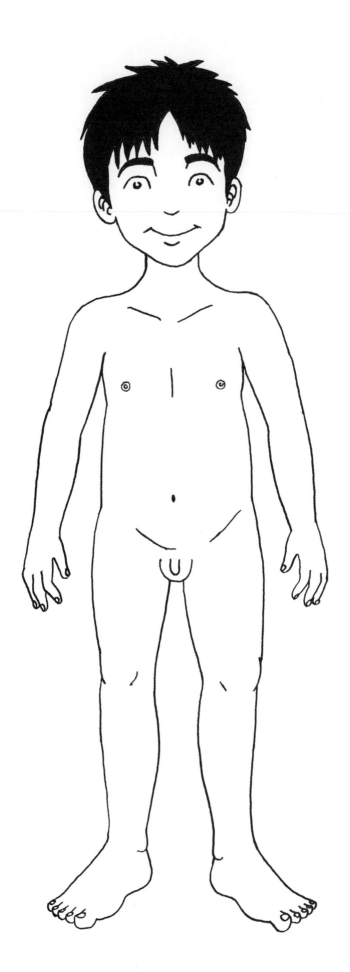

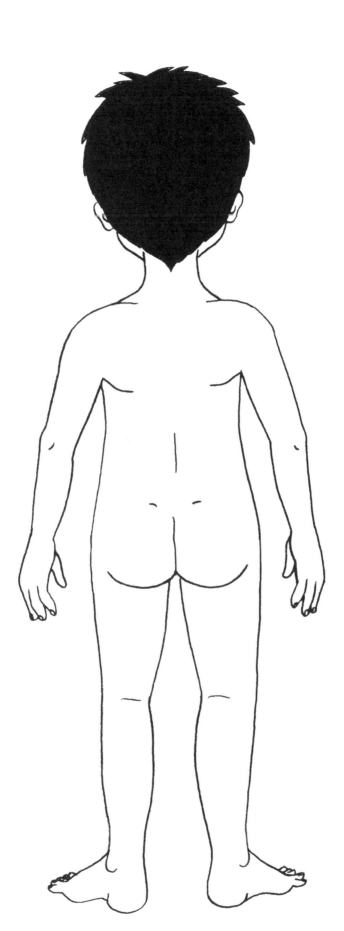

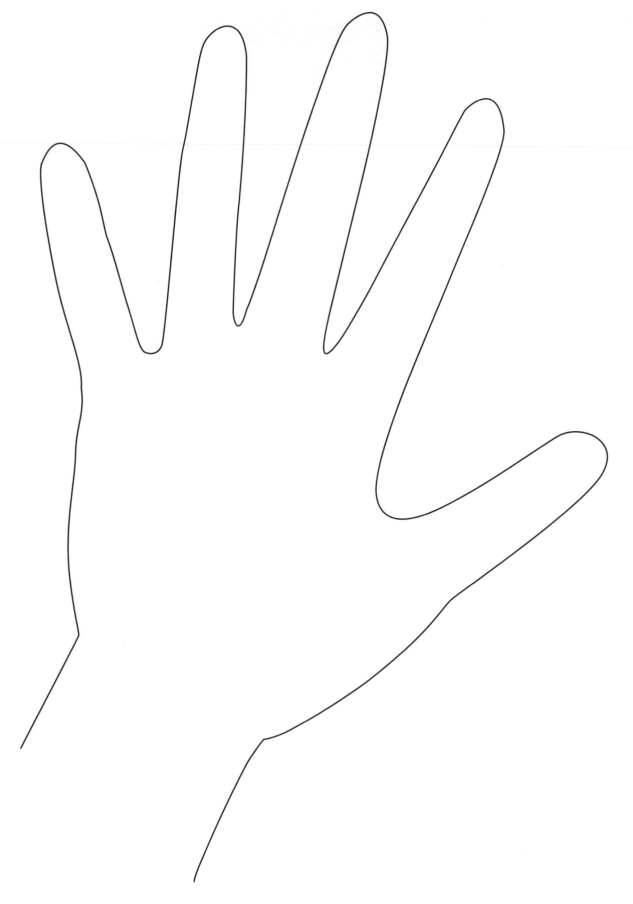

Important information in regards to _____

As an important person to our child, we thank you very much for taking the time to read this letter. We are giving this letter to all the key people in our child's life.

This letter is to inform you that we are educating our child in Body Safety. We wish to empower our child with key Body Safety messages to keep them safe from sexual abuse. Body Safety Education skills and knowledge will assist them to grow into an informed teenager and adult.

From a very young age, we have educated our child in the following key points:

1. We use correct names for all body parts including genitals.

2. Our child knows they are the boss of their body and if they say 'No' to someone coming inside their body boundary then this 'No' needs to be adhered to and respected.

3. Our child knows their private parts are those under their bathing suit.

4. Our child knows not to keep secrets that make them feel bad and/or uncomfortable.

5. Our child knows that no one has the right to touch their private parts, ask them to touch another person's private parts or view images of private parts. If they are asked to do any of these, our child knows to tell a trusted adult on their 'safety network'.

6. Our child knows to keep on telling a person/s on their safety network until they are believed.

7. Our child knows if they are ever touched on their private parts or exposed to images of private parts, it is never ever their fault.

The five people listed below are on our child's safety network. These are the people our child can go to in any unsafe situation and know they will be believed.

We know you will want to work with us to provide the safest possible environment for our child and to reinforce the key points listed above. We thank you very much for caring for our child and helping to keep them safe by respecting and reinforcing the Body Safety messages our child has been taught.

Many thanks

_____

Safety Network

_____

_____

_____

_____

_____

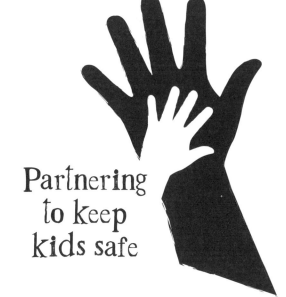

Partnering to keep kids safe

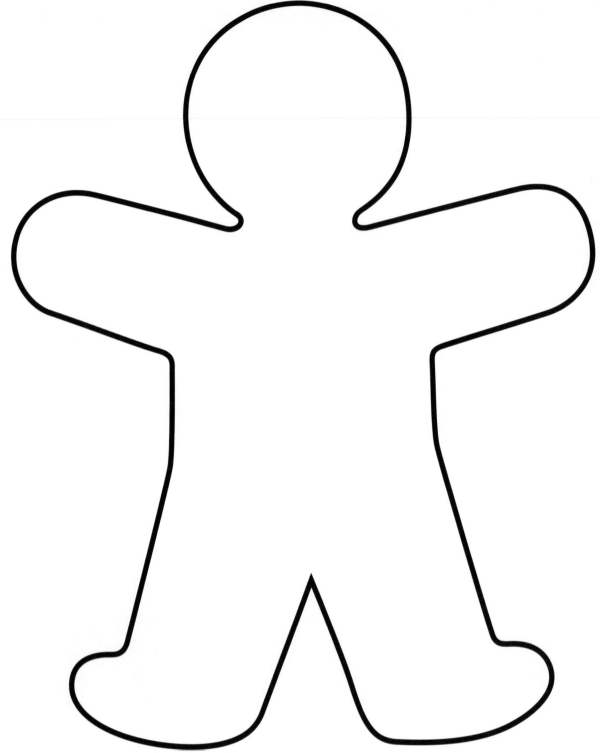

My Body is My Body

Sung to the tune of 'Twinkle Twinkle Little Star'

My body is my body,
And it belongs to me.

No one can touch it
No one but me!

[Point to self]

And if they try,
I'm going to yell, "Stop!"

[Hand comes out to show 'stop']

And run, run, run
As fast as I can,
And yell and tell
Again and again.

[Running motion with arms]

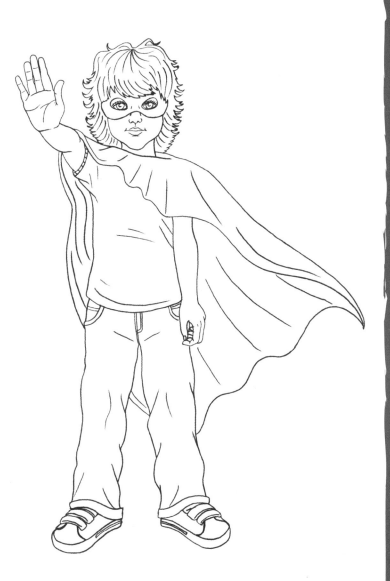

Lyrics by Jayneen Sanders and Debra Byrne

See video at www.e2epublishing.info/body-safety-song/

11

BE LOUD!
BE PROUD!

My Child is Educated in
BODY SAFETY

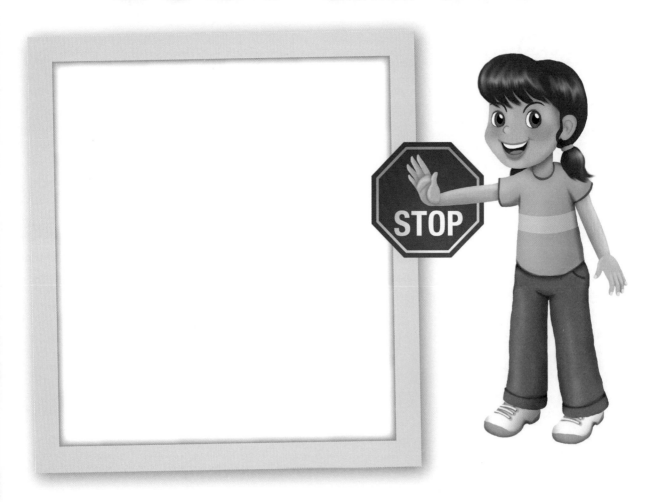

Name: _____

BE LOUD!
BE PROUD!

My Child is Educated in
BODY SAFETY

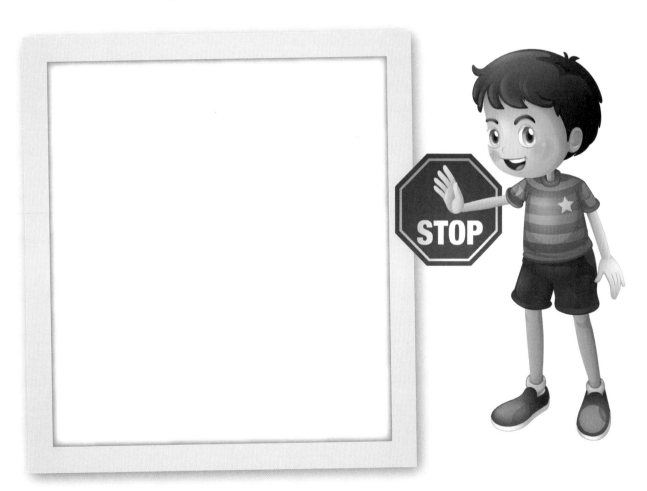

Name: _____

13

"NO!" means "NO!"

I am the Boss of My Body!

Body Safety Education © UpLoad Publishing Pty Ltd 2018
 www.e2epublishing.info

Feelings

Body Safety Skills
Conversation Starter Cards

Please use these Conversation Starter Cards as you see fit and take the conversation where it needs to go. Adapt the conversation starters and language to suit the age of the child. Remember, these are ideas only — you know your child and how best to steer the conversation so the learning is reinforced.

These cards can be used in conjunction with the Key Body Safety Skills outlined on pp. 8–15. They can be used one/two/five at a time. It really is up to you and your child! Use the blank cards for your own conversation starters.

 ## Personal Body Bubble 1

Did you know you have your own personal body bubble around you?

This is your private space and it's just for you!

Can you draw an invisible line around you to show where your personal body bubble goes?

Should anyone enter your personal body bubble if you don't want them to? Why not?

Body Safety Education © UpLoad Publishing Pty Ltd 2018 **www.e2epublishing.info**

 ## Asking Permission

When you go to the dentist, what should the dentist ask you?

Good answer! The dentist should ask if it's okay to look inside your mouth.
He or she should ask your permission.
That means they should ask you if it's okay.

Body Safety Education © UpLoad Publishing Pty Ltd 2018 **www.e2epublishing.info**

Personal Body Bubble 2

What can you do if someone pushes you or comes inside your personal body bubble without you saying it's okay?

That's right! You can say in a strong voice 'No!' or 'Stop!' or 'This is my body bubble/boundary/space and it belongs to me!'

Body Safety Education © UpLoad Publishing Pty Ltd 2018 **www.e2epublishing.info**

 # Consent

When an adult or another child wants to kiss or hug you, and you don't want them to, what can you do?

Yes! You can give the person a high five or a handshake. If you know them quite well, you might like to blow them a kiss.

Body Safety Education © UpLoad Publishing Pty Ltd 2018 **www.e2epublishing.info**

 # Public and Private

What does 'public' mean?

Yes! 'Public' means where there are other people and the space/place is shared by everyone.

What does 'private' mean?

Good answer! 'Private' means just for you.

Body Safety Education © UpLoad Publishing Pty Ltd 2018 **www.e2epublishing.info**

Public Space

Can you name somewhere that is a 'public' space/place?

That's right! The living room is a public space/place because it is shared by everyone. A shopping center is a public space/place, too.

Can you name a public space/place at school?

Awesome answer! The school playground is public space/place because all the students can play there.

Body Safety Education © UpLoad Publishing Pty Ltd 2015   *Some Secrets Should Never Be Kept* **www.e2epublishing.info**

Private Space

Can you name a 'private' space/place or room in your house or at school?

That's right! The toilet is a private space/place in your home and at school. Your bedroom is a private space/place also. You have the right to ask people to not enter your bedroom if you want to be alone and have some privacy.

[Adapt the answer for children who share a bedroom.]

Body Safety Education © UpLoad Publishing Pty Ltd 2018   **www.e2epublishing.info**

Naming Private Parts

Where are your private parts?

You're right! They are the parts of your body that are under your bathing suit.

Can you name your private parts?

That's right! They are your breasts, nipples, bottom/buttocks, penis, vagina, vulva. Your mouth is a private part, too.

[Optional: No one can put anything in your mouth without your permission.]

Body Safety Education © UpLoad Publishing Pty Ltd 2018   **www.e2epublishing.info**

Safety Network

Do you remember what a Safety Network is?

Awesome! It is a group of three to five trusted adults you can tell anything to.

Who are the people on your Safety Network?

Why did you choose those people?

That's right! Because you trust them and they will always believe you when you have something important to tell them.

Body Safety Education © UpLoad Publishing Pty Ltd 2018 **www.e2epublishing.info**

Unsafe Touch

Should anyone touch your private parts?

What must you do if someone does touch your private parts?

Yes! You must tell an adult on your Safety Network straightaway.

You can also put out your hand like this and say 'No!' to that person and then GO very quickly and TELL! TELL! TELL!

Body Safety Education © UpLoad Publishing Pty Ltd 2018 **www.e2epublishing.info**

Unsafe Secrets 1

What would you do if an older child or adult touched your private parts and they told you to keep it a secret? *Good job! You must tell an adult on your Safety Network straightaway and you must keep on telling until you are believed.*

But what if the person said that if you tell the secret they will do something bad to your mother/pet; should you STILL tell the secret? What if they say no one will believe you; should you STILL tell the secret? *Exactly right! You must STILL tell an adult on your Safety Network straightaway. You must Tell! Tell! Tell!*

Body Safety Education © UpLoad Publishing Pty Ltd 2018 **www.e2epublishing.info**

Early Warning Signs

What are your Early Warning Signs?
That's right! You might have sweaty palms, shaky legs, a sick feeling in your tummy and you may feel like crying.

Have you ever felt your Early Warning Signs?

What happened to make you feel this way?

What did you do?

Great job! You told someone on your Safety Network.

Body Safety Education © UpLoad Publishing Pty Ltd 2015   *Some Secrets Should Never Be Kept* **www.e2epublishing.info**

 # Saying 'No!'

Are you allowed to say 'No!' to an adult or older child?
Great answer! You can certainly say 'No!' if they are doing something that you don't like or that brings on your Early Warning Signs.

Do you remember what your Early Warning Signs are?
Correct! You may get sweaty palms, a racing heart and feel sick in your tummy. You might also get shaky legs and a headache.

What other things might happen to your body when you get your Early Warning Signs?

Body Safety Education © UpLoad Publishing Pty Ltd 2018   **www.e2epublishing.info**

 # Feelings

How do you feel if someone pushes you over?

How do you feel when you are playing in the park with a friend?

How do you feel at the top of a big slide for the first time?

How do you feel on your birthday?

[Extend the child's answers, e.g. by asking, Why do you feel…?
What do you mean when you say…? Where do you feel this in your body?]

Body Safety Education © UpLoad Publishing Pty Ltd 2018   **www.e2epublishing.info**

Feelings — Safe/Unsafe

When do you feel safe?

Tell me about a time/s when you felt safe/unsafe?

Do you feel safe tucked up in bed? Why? Why not?

Do you feel safe near an angry, barking dog? Why not?

Body Safety Education © UpLoad Publishing Pty Ltd 2018 **www.e2epublishing.info**

 # Feelings — Angry/Sad

How do you feel when you are angry?

Where do you feel this in your body?

What makes you feel angry?

How do you feel when you are sad?

Where do you feel this in your body?

What makes you feel sad?

Body Safety Education © UpLoad Publishing Pty Ltd 2018 **www.e2epublishing.info**

 # Feelings — Happy

How do you feel when you are happy?

Where do you feel this in your body?

What makes you feel happy?

Are you happy every day?

What makes you feel unhappy?

Body Safety Education © UpLoad Publishing Pty Ltd 2018 **www.e2epublishing.info**

Feelings — Scared

Do you feel scared sometimes?

When do you feel scared?

Where do you feel this in your body?

What can you do if you feel scared?

Body Safety Education © UpLoad Publishing Pty Ltd 2015   *Some Secrets Should Never Be Kept* **www.e2epublishing.info**

Happy Secrets/Surprises

Can you keep a happy secret/surprise, such as not telling your grandmother about a special birthday present? Why? Why not?

Can you name me some happy secrets/surprises?

Why are they happy secrets/surprises?

Yes! Because they will be told very soon.

Body Safety Education © UpLoad Publishing Pty Ltd 2018   **www.e2epublishing.info**

Unsafe Secrets 2

Imagine someone gave you some special sweets and told you to keep them a secret. Should you keep that kind of secret?

What should you say to the person asking you to keep that kind of secret?

Awesome! You could say clearly and in a strong voice that you don't keep those kinds of secrets, and that you only keep happy surprises that will be told soon.

Body Safety Education © UpLoad Publishing Pty Ltd 2018   **www.e2epublishing.info**

Body Safety Education © UpLoad Publishing Pty Ltd 2018
May be photocopied for non-commercial use.   **www.e2epublishing.info**

Unsafe Secrets 3

Should you keep secrets that make you feel bad and uncomfortable?

What should you do if you are asked to keep that kind of secret?

That's right! You must tell an adult on your Safety Network straightaway.

Have you ever kept a secret that made you feel bad and uncomfortable?

What did you do?

Body Safety Education © UpLoad Publishing Pty Ltd 2018 **www.e2epublishing.info**

 # Unsafe Secrets 4

What should you do if you are shown or you see pictures of private parts?

Yes! You should tell a trusted adult on your Safety Network straightaway.

Should you keep a secret about seeing pictures of people's private parts?

Good answer! You should NEVER keep that kind of secret. You must tell an adult on your Safety Network straightaway.

Body Safety Education © UpLoad Publishing Pty Ltd 2018 **www.e2epublishing.info**

 # Private Parts 1

When might it be okay for an adult to touch your private parts?

That's right! If a doctor or nurse needs to look at your private parts because you are unwell BUT only when a trusted adult is with you.

Of course, when we are babies our parents (caregivers) need to wash and dry our private parts but as we get older, we can do this by ourselves.

Body Safety Education © UpLoad Publishing Pty Ltd 2018 **www.e2epublishing.info**

Private Parts 2

Sometimes we can be touched on our private parts and it feels good, but our Early Warning Signs still happen to us. This can be confusing, but remember even if the touch feels good, no one should touch your private parts in that way.

What should you do if this happens to you?

Exactly! You should tell a trusted adult on your Safety Network straightaway.

Body Safety Education © UpLoad Publishing Pty Ltd 2015   *Some Secrets Should Never Be Kept* **www.e2epublishing.info**

Private Parts 3

Can you touch your own private parts?

Yes, you're right! You can! But only in a private space/place.

When might you need to touch your private parts?

That's right! When you are washing your private parts in the bath or shower, or when you are using the toilet.

Body Safety Education © UpLoad Publishing Pty Ltd 2018   **www.e2epublishing.info**

Body Safety Education © UpLoad Publishing Pty Ltd 2018
May be photocopied for non-commercial use.   **www.e2epublishing.info**

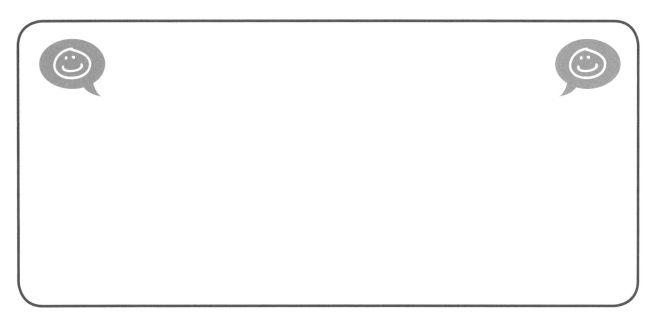

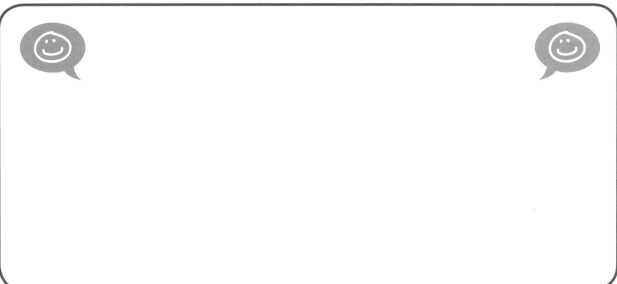

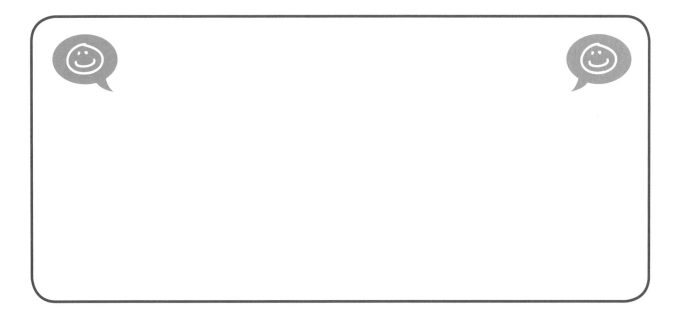

Notes